HERBAL ANTIBIOTICS REVOLUTION

Exploring The Potency Of Herbal Antibiotics For Holistic Health.

By

Stephanie Mejorado

Table Of Contents

Introduction.

Discover the game-changing ***Herbal Antibiotics Revolution*** and how it can improve your health in every way. When ancient herbal wisdom meets modern medical science, you will experience the restorative power of nature. *Embrace a holistic approach to health where potent plants can strengthen your immune system and promote overall vitality.* Join the effort to learn about herbal antibiotics and help create a healthier, more sustainable future.

This article presents a very fast account of the history of ***Antibiotics***, covering the period from the discovery of the first antibiotics to the current state of things, which is marked by the growth of numerous antibiotic-resistant illnesses that are difficult to cure. The concerns of antibiotic resistance are addressed in a number of ways, including the invention of innovative methods for the quest for novel antimicrobials, the construction of more potent preventive measures, and—above all—a greater grasp of the ecology of antibiotics and antibiotic resistance. Also explored is the enlargement of conceptual frameworks in view of modern breakthroughs in the disciplines of chemotherapy, antibiotic resistance, and antimicrobials.

Prior to getting started, let's quickly clarify: **Antibiotics: what are they?**

By destroying bacteria or limiting their growth within the body, antibiotics treat bacterial infections. Antibiotics can be injected intravenously, topically *(cream, ointment, spray),* **orally** *(pills, capsules, liquids).*

For mild illnesses, lung infections, ear infections, and sore throats, antibiotics are not routinely prescribed. Furthermore, viral infections, such as the common cold and influenza, cannot be treated with antibiotics. *Antibiotic resistance may occur from inappropriate or overused antibiotics.* Antibiotic-resistant bacteria cause roughly 2 million illnesses and many fatalities in the United States each year.

Antibiotics' Past

One of the leading causes of illness and mortality in the human population was infectious illness. In *Serbia, China, Greece, and Egypt,* microorganisms that generate antibiotics were exploited as interventions to treat infectious diseases prior to the commencement of the modern antibiotic era, which happened more than *2000* years ago. The first reference to moldy bread and medicinal soils being used to alleviate ailments is recorded in the Ebers papyrus, an Egyptian medical papyrus dated 1550 BC. Similar to this, human bones discovered from the Dakhleh Oasis in Egypt found signs of the chelating antibody tetracycline.

When Do We Use Antibiotics?

Here are the simple step on how to treat bacterial infection through antibiotics:

- Are unlikely to go away in the absence of antibiotics.

- Might spread to others if left untreated.

- It might take too long to resolve if therapy is not received.

- Pose a danger of developing more serious complications.

Chapter 1: A Challenging Strategy For Comprehending Bacteria In Herbs.

The scientific community has long been captivated by the complicated interplay between bacteria and herbs, which presents a puzzle that is difficult to answer. As we strive to grasp the complicated interactions between these two domains, a tough approach becomes apparent—one that demands a multidisciplinary vision, inventive tactics, and a commitment to go against the grain. *We can learn more about the probable medical benefits of herbs and how they interact with bacterial illnesses by acknowledging this complexity.*

Important Components Of The Challenging Approach:

Deciphering The Microbial Ecosystem

The complex microbial populations that exist in herbs are a challenging conundrum to solve. In order to address this, powerful metagenomic and metatranscriptomic approaches can be applied to examine the complicated microbial ecosystems found in herbs. We can learn more about the diversity, connections, and functional roles of both dangerous and good bacteria by sequencing and studying the genetic material of these microbial communities. With the use of this approach, we will be able to interpret the intricate network of microbial interactions present in herbs, providing insight into how these communities affect the general well-being and features of the plants. Furthermore, analyzing the spatial distribution of these microbial communities within the plant tissues as well as how they react to external stimuli can shed light on how dynamic the relationship between the microorganisms and the herb is. With the aid of state-of-the-art molecular biology and bioinformatics approaches, we may unravel the mysteries of these complex microbial communities and open the way to a deeper comprehension of bacteria in herbs.

✓. Molecular Interactions that Are Dynamic: It involves an interdisciplinary approach that integrates advanced molecular biology, bioinformatics, and ecology principles to understand the dynamic interactions at the molecular level within herb microbial communities. *Using metagenomic technologies to sequence and study the genetic material of the microbial communities related to herbs is a vital step.* With the use of metagenomic analysis, the great diversity of bacterial species that are present can be identified, as can their putative activities, including the genes in charge of nutrient cycling, stimulating plant development, and suppressing diseases.

Moreover, the analysis of metatranscriptomics can offer valuable perspectives on the gene expression profiles of these microbial communities, clarifying their functional functions and reactivity to external stimuli. With this technology, we can appreciate how molecular interactions occur between microbial populations and the host plant and how they dynamically react to changes in their environment.

Apart from genetic and transcriptional research, one can see the geographical distribution of particular microbial species within plant tissues by applying spatial mapping techniques like fluorescence in situ hybridization *(FISH)* and in situ hybridization (*ISH*). The location of helpful bacteria, probable pathogen hotspots, and the general composition of the plant's microbial population can all be found utilizing this geographical data.

Furthermore, combining genetic data with ecological concepts like niche differentiation and community dynamics can offer a thorough insight into the interactions that occur among herbivore microbial populations. For example, analyzing the reactions of microbial communities to environmental cues like temperature, moisture content, and soil type might illuminate the ecological mechanisms impacting these connections.

Ultimately, we can comprehend the intricate network of dynamic molecular interactions between herbs and the microbial communities they are linked to by integrating multiple approaches. This complete understanding will increase our understanding of the interactions between herbs and bacteria and have repercussions for herbal medicine, sustainable agriculture, and ecosystem management.

✓. Integrating Conventional Knowledge with Contemporary Science:

Combining the behaviors, knowledge, and ideas from antiquated cultures with the most recent scientific discoveries entails uniting traditional wisdom with modern science to provide a comprehensive and all-encompassing strategy for dealing with a range of issues. A framework for implementing this integration is offered here:

✓. Respect and Preservation of Traditional Knowledge:

Appreciate the relevance of indigenous knowledge systems and traditional wisdom. Recognize the tremendous wisdom inherited from previous generations regarding ecosystems, medicinal plants, and natural resources.

✓. **Documentation and Validation:** Work collaboratively to record traditional knowledge and practices with communities and practitioners. Next, apply contemporary scientific tools like field research, lab analysis, and clinical trials to verify these conventional assumptions.

✓. **Ethnobotanical and Ethnopharmacological Studies:** To identify plants and natural products used in traditional medical systems, conduct ethnobotanical and ethnopharmacological research. This requires examining these natural remedies' probable therapeutic effects as well as their traditional use and preparation processes.

✓. Bioprospecting and Drug Development: Examine conventionally used medical plants and chemicals to discover whether they have any use in the quest for novel medications. This comprises the isolation of bioactive compounds, the discovery of their mechanisms of action, and the rigorous scientific assessment of their safety and effectiveness.

✓. **Cultural Sensitivity and Collaboration:** Treat indigenous populations, community leaders, and traditional healers with respect and care for their cultural traditions. Encourage cooperative alliances that respect conventional wisdom and merge it with contemporary scientific techniques.

✓. **Integrative Medicine:** Create integrative healthcare solutions that integrate current medical treatments with age-old healing methods. This may mean incorporating complementary therapies such as herbal medications, acupuncture, meditation, and others into established healthcare systems.

✓. Conservation and Sustainable Use: Strive to maintain natural resources and conventionally used medicinal plants in a sustainable manner. Encourage conservation projects to save traditional places, biodiversity, and the cultural legacy associated with conventional medical treatments.

✓. Education and Awareness: Spread the word about the importance of traditional knowledge systems and encourage people to learn about them. To enhance respect and understanding amongst traditional practitioners, scientists, policymakers, and the general public, stimulate dialog.

✓. **Policy Development and Legal Protection:** Promote legislation that acknowledges and defends cultural heritage, traditional knowledge, and intellectual property rights. Involve traditional communities in decision-making processes that affect their resources and skills.

Healthcare, conservation, and sustainable resource management can all benefit from a more all-encompassing and inclusive approach that integrates the wisdom of old practices with the rigor of contemporary scientific investigation. Global society as a whole, as well as traditional communities, stand to gain from this integration.

Cultural Sensitivity and Ethical Issues:

Integrating ancient knowledge with contemporary study requires careful consideration of ethical issues and cultural sensitivity. *Here's how to tackle these elements:*

• **Respect for Indigenous Rights:** Acknowledge and uphold the rights of indigenous groups to their natural resources, customs, and traditional knowledge. Give their sovereignty, autonomy, and right to self-determination first priority in any cooperative endeavors.

• **Informed Consent:** Before undertaking a study or making use of traditional practitioners' or community members' skills, seek their informed consent. Make sure that everyone knows and agrees to engage in the collaboration by fully defining its aims, prospective advantages, and risks.

• **Benefit Sharing:** To assure that traditional communities obtain genuine advantages from the commercialization or use of their resources and expertise, fair and equitable benefit-sharing processes should be implemented. This could comprise initiatives for capacity-building, revenue sharing, or other sorts of compensation.

• **Protection of Intellectual Property:** Use ethical norms and legal safeguards to conserve traditional knowledge and cultural manifestations. Observe customary rights to intellectual property and promote actions aimed at limiting the exploitation or theft of indigenous knowledge.

• **Cultural Appropriateness:** Make sure that collaborative efforts, scientific research methodology, and communication tactics respect and are compatible with traditional customs, beliefs, and values. Modify research methodologies to conform to the customs and cultural norms of the place.

• **Community Engagement and Participation:** Include people of the community, elders, and traditional healers in all phases of the research process, from project idea to execution and findings distribution. Encourage meaningful engagement and knowledge co-creation.

• Cultural Competency Training:
To strengthen the cultural
competency and comprehension of
traditional knowledge systems of
academics, healthcare practitioners,
and other stakeholders, provide
training and capacity-building
opportunities.

• Language and Communication:
Honor the transfer of information
through oral traditions and native
languages. To enhance fruitful
discussion and comprehension, utilize
basic, approachable language and

culturally appropriate communication approaches.

- **Conflict Resolution:** Provide processes for addressing disagreements or conflicts that can occur between researchers, traditional practitioners, and other interested parties. Provide explicit mechanisms for addressing disagreements and sustaining moral norms.

- **Long-Term Relationships:** Build respectful, reciprocal, and trusting connections with traditional communities that will benefit both sides over the long haul. Beyond the short-term goals of the research, vow to continue communication, cooperation, and support for community needs.

It is possible to guarantee that the process of fusing traditional wisdom with contemporary science is carried out in a responsible, courteous, and inclusive way that respects the various cultures and knowledge systems involved by incorporating these ethical considerations and cultural sensitivity principles into the process.

Although grasping microorganisms in herbs through a complicated technique is a demanding task, there are major rewards that could lead to both scientific comprehension and potential therapeutic purposes. We can start a revolutionary path toward understanding the hidden link between bacteria and herbs by embracing complexity, integrating multiple viewpoints, and expanding the bounds of present knowledge. By doing this, we might unearth ground-breaking discoveries that could affect the course of biotechnology and healthcare in the future.

Chapter 2: **Antibiotics Cure.**

Certain kinds of bacterial infections are treated or prevented with the use of antibiotics. *They destroy bacteria or inhibit them from growing and expanding.* Viral infections cannot be treated with antibiotics. This covers

the majority of coughs, sore throats,
the common cold, and the flu.

Moreover, it is occasionally taken as
a prophylactic strategy against
infection. Antibiotic prophylaxis is
the phrase used for this.

Operation:

- Prophylactic antibiotic treatment
  is often indicated if you are
  having surgery in a particular
  place. This is due to the
  likelihood of an increased risk of
  infection.

- You can find out from your surgical team whether you require antibiotic prophylaxis.

- In addition, antibiotic prophylaxis could be indicated for recurrent illnesses such as:

Infection With Bacteria.

1. A bacterial skin infection termed cellulitis usually affects the skin's deeper layers. It is usually brought on by bacteria, either Streptococcus or

Staphylococcus, seeping into the skin through a cut, crack, or other hole in the epidermis. The afflicted region becomes painful, swollen, and red.

2. The indicators of the infection can include warmth, pain, and even fever, and they can spread swiftly. A specialist in healthcare should prescribe antibiotics for the quick treatment of cellulitis. If you suspect you may have cellulitis, you must consult a doctor right away because untreated cases can have hazardous side effects.

3. Cellulitis can be avoided by following basic hygiene, attending to cuts on the skin right away, and taking care of underlying disorders that damage the immune system.

An Infection Of The Urinary Tract.

An infection in the kidneys, bladder, urethra, or any other region of the urinary system.
Women develop urinary tract infections more commonly. Most typically, they attack the bladder or urethra, but more serious infections involve the kidney.

UTI *risk factors include sexual activity, abnormalities of the urinary tract, immune system suppression, and the use of certain contraceptives. Antibiotics, greater fluid consumption, and lifestyle adjustments are generally part of the treatment.*

Kidney infections are among the more dangerous side effects of untreated UTIs. It's vital to receive medical care as soon as you feel you may have a UTI.

Herpes Genital.

One form of sexually transmitted infection *(STI)* is genital herpes.

Herpetic sores are unpleasant blisters *(fluid-filled lumps)* that have the potential to burst open and discharge fluid.

Reasons for vaginal herpes
There are two types of herpes that cause genital herpes. *simplex virus (HSV):*

1. HSV-1. Although genital herpes can also arise from this kind, cold sores are frequently the result.

2. HSV-2. This variety can result in cold sores in addition to the typical genital herpes.

✓. **Primary Infection:** Flu-like symptoms and painful sores. Repeated Events: mild symptoms with intermittent flare-ups. Transfer:

✓. **Sexual Contact:** Sexual activity is the primary route to spreading.

Vertical Transmission: During childbirth, a mother may transmit an infection to her newborn.

Diagnose And Therapy.

Testing: by PCR, blood testing, or swabs.
Antiviral drugs regulate symptoms and lower the incidence of viral infections.
No Cure: Antivirals can manage symptoms, but there is no proven cure for herpes.

Avoidance:

- Condoms are not perfect, but they do offer some protection.

- Steer clear of contact during outbreaks. When an outbreak is active, the danger of transmission is greatest.

Effect:

✓. **Emotional Strain:** The stigma linked to herpes can cause emotional difficulties.

Complications: *may boost the possibility of developing or spreading HIV.*

Getting medical help is vital for an accurate diagnosis and treatment. Managing genital herpes needs regular communication with sexual partners, safe sex techniques, and an understanding of the hazards.

Fever With Rheumatism.

The development of rheumatic fever commonly begins two to four weeks following a strep throat infection.

Swelling, also known as inflammation, in the skin, joints, heart, or central nervous system causes symptoms. There might be one or more symptoms. A person suffering from rheumatic fever may experience intermittent or changing symptoms.

Symptoms Of Rheumatic Fever Can Include:

A fever. Swelling or pain in the joints, notably in the knees, ankles, elbows, and wrists.

Joints could feel achy or hot. a discomfort radiating from one joint to another.

Aching in the chest. small, painless protuberances under the skin. Roughly edged, painless rash that is either flat or slightly raised.

Sydenham chorea is a disease that certain rheumatic fever sufferers encounter. This condition's symptoms include:

Uncontrollable, jerky movements of the hands, feet, and face are prevalent.

Crying fits or inappropriate laughter fits.

Chapter 3: 10 Types Of Herbal Antibiotics.

What are the ten herbal antibiotics that are most frequently used?

Ten common kinds of antibiotics are given below:

1. Penicillins.

These are widely applied to treat a range of infections, such as:

urinary tract infections, skin infections, and chest infections

2.Cephalosporins.

These are useful against a number of infections. Certain ones are also beneficial in treating infections that are more serious, such as:

meningitis, septicemia

3.Aminoglycosides.

A class of drugs called aminoglycosides is used to treat diverse bacterial infections. Among these are drugs such as tobramycin, amikacin, and gentamicin. These antibiotics function by blocking the synthesis of proteins by bacteria, which affects bacterial cell functioning and finally ends in cell death.

Protein synthesis is impeded by the route of action, which involves binding to the bacterial ribosome and, more notably, to the 30S subunit. This disruption works especially well against gram-negative, aerobic bacteria. Aminoglycosides are typically used for severe infections or in instances where other antibiotics might not perform as well.

Aminoglycosides can cause substantial side effects, including potential renal and inner ear damage, despite their effectiveness. To reduce toxicity while increasing therapeutic effects, blood level monitoring is necessary. Because of their limited oral absorption, these antibiotics are frequently administered intravenously or intramuscularly.

In conclusion, aminoglycosides are potent antibiotics that operate against certain infections by inhibiting bacteria from making proteins. To control any probable harmful outcomes, though, close supervision is important.

4.Tetracyclines.

One class of antibiotics called tetracyclines stops bacteria from producing proteins. *They function by binding themselves to the bacterial ribosome and blocking aminoacyl-tRNA from joining the mRNA-ribosome complex.* This interference inhibits the growing peptide chain during protein synthesis from elongating, which in turn slows the growth of bacteria.

Broad-spectrum antibiotics like tetracyclines perform well against a variety of bacteria, including Gram-positive and Gram-negative. They are frequently used to treat a number of ailments, including cutaneous, respiratory, and urinary tract infections. Bacterial resistance has, however, occasionally hampered their potency.

It's crucial to understand that tetracyclines could induce adverse effects such as photosensitivity and gastrointestinal difficulties. Furthermore, due to their possible harmful effects on growing teeth and bones, their consumption may be limited in particular populations, such as kids and pregnant women. Like with any antibiotic, appropriate use and following dosage requirements are vital to prevent resistance and guarantee good treatment.

5. Macrolides.

These antibiotics belong to a class that is differentiated by a macrocyclic lactone ring. Clarithromycin, azithromycin, and erythromycin are classic examples. By binding to the bacterial ribosome's 50S component and inhibiting the synthesis of peptide bonds, they limit the manufacturing of proteins in bacteria.

✓. **Mechanism of Action:** By binding to the bacterial ribosome's 50S component, macrolides impede the creation of proteins by bacteria. The peptide chain cannot elongate during translation because this binding inhibits the translocation step.

✓. **Range of Action:** Macrolides have a broad anti-gram-positive bacterial spectrum that includes

Staphylococcus aureus and Streptococcus pneumoniae. Additionally, they exhibit some effects against atypical illnesses and certain Gram-negative bacteria.

✓. **Clinical Uses:** Macrolides are widely used to treat infections of the skin and soft tissues, infections of the respiratory system, and various illnesses that are transmitted through sexual activity. They are widely viewed as a replacement for people with penicillin allergies.

✓. **Pharmacokinetics:** Macrolides normally permeate tissues well and are well absorbed when administered orally. For instance, azithromycin's prolonged half-life enables a once-daily dose.

✓. *Side Effects:* Gastrointestinal problems, including nausea and diarrhea, are frequently observed as side effects. Additionally, macrolides could lengthen the QT interval, which, in vulnerable patients, might result in arrhythmias.

✓. **Drug Interactions:** By stimulating or inhibiting cytochrome P450 enzymes, macrolides can interact with other drugs. This may change how different medications are digested, perhaps leading to interactions.

✓. **Resistance:** Modification of the target site on the ribosome or efflux pumps are two mechanisms that might lead to bacterial resistance to macrolides.

Antibiotics known as macrolides function by blocking the synthesis of bacterial proteins, which makes them effective against a wide spectrum of infections, notably those brought on by Gram-positive bacteria. It is vital for their effective and safe utilization in medical practice to know their mechanism of action, clinical applications, and potential side effects.

6.Monobactams.

A beta-lactam ring makes up the characteristic chemical structure of monobactams, a class of antibiotics. Monobactam antibiotics have a single lactam ring in their structure, in contrast to other beta-lactam antibiotics such as cephalosporins and penicillins.

Aztreonam is one well-known example of a monobactam. A wide spectrum of Gram-negative bacteria, even those resistant to other beta-lactam antibiotics, can be efficiently combated with aztreonam. Because it can elude beta-lactamases, which are bacterial enzymes that can break down beta-lactam rings and render antibiotics worthless, it is limited to Gram-negative bacteria.

When treating infections brought on by Gram-negative bacteria, monobactam antibiotics are crucial, especially when resistance to conventional antibiotics is a worry. Monobactams' particular mechanism of action and decreased cross-reactivity with other beta-lactam antibiotics are enabled by their different structures.

7. The Carbapenems.

A class of broad-spectrum antibiotics called carbapenems is used to treat a variety of bacterial diseases. They share structural similarities with penicillin and are classified as beta-lactam antibiotics. Imipenem, meropenem, doripenem, and ertapenem are classic examples.

These antibiotics function by blocking the production of the bacterial cell wall, which prevents the formation of peptidoglycan, a key component of the bacterial cell wall, from occurring. Compared to other beta-lactam antibiotics, carbapenems demonstrate a larger spectrum of activity, rendering them efficacious against a diverse array of bacteria, spanning both gram-positive and gram-negative strains.

The resilience of carbapenems against multiple beta-lactamases, which are enzymes produced by some bacteria to break down beta-lactam antibiotics, is one of their notable qualities. However, a major difficulty in hospital settings is the generation of carbapenem-resistant kinds of bacteria, which are typically produced by the production of carbapenemases.

It's vital to use carbapenems sparingly in order to stop the evolution of antibiotic resistance. When other, less potent antibiotics are either ineffective or inappropriate, these medications are normally saved for more serious diseases.

8.   Fluoroquinolones.

The broad-spectrum systemic antibacterial fluoroquinolones are a family of medications that have been widely utilized to treat urinary tract and respiratory infections. The vast spectrum of aerobic gram-positive and gram-negative organisms is vulnerable to the action of fluoroquinolones.

Levofloxacin, moxifloxacin, and ciprofloxacin are a few examples. Although they operate well against a wide spectrum of germs, their application is often limited to serious infections because of the likelihood of side effects such as tendinitis, a torn tendon, and effects on the central nervous system.

Fluoroquinolones must be used carefully, taking into account the risk-benefit ratio and the likelihood of antibiotic resistance. It is vital to contact a healthcare expert to ensure proper use and avoid unwanted effects.

9. The Sulfonamides.

Sulphonamides are a key class of antibiotics with a broad spectrum of action that operate exceedingly effectively against both gram-positive and certain gram-negative bacteria.

It's also one of the oldest and most frequently used antibiotics. Despite being mostly overtaken by newer antibiotics because of side effects and resistance difficulties, they are nevertheless helpful in specific medical applications. For a variety of bacterial infections, trimethoprim-sulfamethoxazole—a combination of a sulfonamide and another antibiotic—is routinely administered.

10. The Trimethoprim.

An antibiotic called trimethoprim is used to treat bacterial infections. It operates by preventing bacterial growth.

It is a member of the
dihydrofolate reductase inhibitor
pharmacological class. In order
for tetrahydrofolate to be
generated, which is necessary for
the production of *DNA, RNA,*
and proteins in bacteria, an
enzyme known as dihydrofolate
reductase must be blocked by
trimethoprim.

Trimethoprim interferes with the
metabolism of folate, which
stops the bacterial cell from
multiplying and reproducing. It
frequently works synergistically
with sulfamethoxazole
(TMP-SMX, or Bactrim) by

focusing on distinct stages of the folate synthesis pathway and improving their combined antibacterial activity.

- For bacterial infections of the respiratory, urinary, and other systems, trimethoprim is routinely used. Although it is normally well received, it can have adverse effects like any other medication, including allergic reactions or gastrointestinal difficulties. To guarantee effective treatment and reduce the possibility of antibiotic resistance, trimethoprim must only be used

as advised by a healthcare
provider, just like any other
antibiotic.

Chapter 4: **Startling Statistics About Alternative Medicine.**

Any medical technique that is not considered standard practice in Western medicine is often referred to as "alternative therapy." Alternative medicine is the phrase used to describe methods that are utilized in addition to standard medical procedures.

Beyond that, the field of complementary and alternative

medicines is so diverse that it is challenging to identify them. It comprises, among other things, hypnosis, chiropractic adjustments, modifications in food and exercise, and putting needles into the skin *(also known as acupuncture).*

There is substantial discussion concerning the advantages of alternative therapy. Even though further research is required to determine the usefulness of practically all of these strategies, people are continuously experimenting with them.

These are a handful of the approaches that are influencing how people view health care.

All About Natural Medicine.

Naturopathic medicine is a vast category of alternative medicine that is based on the notion that nature has the potential to cure.

Both conventional and complementary medicine are taught to naturopathic physicians. By evaluating a condition's mental, physiological, and spiritual manifestations in a particular patient, they try to uncover the underlying cause of the sickness.

A multitude of therapeutic techniques are often utilized in naturopathy, such as acupuncture, homeopathy, herbal therapy, behavioral adjustments, and nutrition.

Ten truths regarding alternative medicine in the present world.

Alternative medical treatments have existed for countless years.

People have been adopting alternative healing techniques for thousands of years to boost their health and well-being instead of relying entirely on conventional Western medicine. *These treatments, which include energy healing and herbal medications, have risen in popularity recently.* These are ten things you might not be aware of about alternative medicine in the present world.

Over one-third of Americans receive alternative medical treatment.

Alternative medicine has been practiced all over the world for thousands of years. For example, Ayurvedic medicine, which has its roots in India, has been used for over 5,000 years, and traditional Chinese medicine has been used for over 2,500 years.

✓. Addiction Therapy With Acupuncture.

Over one-third of Americans utilize alternative therapies, with herbal supplements, chiropractic adjustments, and yoga being the most popular, according to the National Center for Complementary and Integrative Health.

✓. Aromatherapy Can Reduce Tension And Enhance Mood.

It has been revealed that acupuncture, an ancient Chinese medical method that involves placing needles in precise body areas, is useful in the treatment of addiction. Withdrawal symptoms and cravings might be minimized for people in recovery from substance addiction.

✓. Reiki Helps Facilitate Healing And Minimize Discomfort.

It has been established that aromatherapy, which uses essential oils to improve mood and stimulate relaxation, is useful in relieving stress and anxiety. Some oils, like chamomile and lavender, are widely known for their soothing properties.

✓. Homeopathy Heals Ailments With Highly Diluted Substances.

It has been established that Reiki, a sort of energy healing that requires manipulating the body's energy fields with the hands, is beneficial for alleviating pain and expediting healing. It frequently serves as a complement to standard medical care.

✓. Reflexology Can Relieve Discomfort And Enhance Circulation.

As an alternative medicinal technique, homeopathy treats ailments with extremely diluted substances. Homeopathy operates on the idea that the body is capable of self-healing and that the highly diluted chemicals aid in this process.

✓. Yoga Can Promote Balance, Strength, And Flexibility.

It has been established that reflexology, a technique that entails applying pressure to particular regions on the hands, feet, and ears, is good for increasing circulation and lowering discomfort. It is widely used as an adjuvant treatment for conditions like migraines and arthritis.

✓. Tai Chi Can Aid Older Adults With Their Balance And Prevent Falls.

It has been discovered that yoga, a sort of physical posture, breathing methods, and meditation, is excellent for developing flexibility, strength, and balance. Additionally, it can alleviate tension and increase relaxation.

✓. Meditation Can Relieve Anxiety And Enhance Mental Health.

Tai Chi is a slow-moving, flowing Chinese martial art that has been demonstrated to assist older adults' balance and minimize their chance of falling. It can ease stress and encourage adaptability.

It has been established that meditation, a practice that involves quieting the mind and focusing on

*one's thoughts, is useful for
increasing mental health and
lowering anxiety. Additionally, it can
boost concentration and focus.*

In summary, complementary and
alternative medicine has a rich history
and presents a diversity of
advantages. They can give consumers
a more complete approach to
wellbeing and support conventional
medical procedures. Although some
people may not benefit from
alternative treatment methods, it's still
vital to be open-minded and
investigate all of your options if you

want the finest possible health and
fitness.

Chapter 5: Antibacterial Usage: All You Should Know.

Antibacterials are substances that either eliminate or stop bacteria from multiplying. They are crucial to medicine, mostly in the treatment of bacterial infections. Here's a basic rundown:

Antibacterial Types.

Antibiotics are compounds that are either synthetically made to target bacteria or obtained from biological entities such as fungi and bacteria.

Antiseptics are used on living tissues to prevent or destroy the growth of bacteria.

Disinfectants are used to eradicate bacteria from surfaces or inanimate things.

Applications:

<> **Medical Treatment:** To treat bacterial infections in humans, physicians prescribe antibiotics.

<> **Preventive measures:** Using prophylactic medication in some cases, notably before surgery, can help avoid infections.

<> **Hygiene Practices:** To keep homes and healthcare facilities clean, antiseptics and disinfectants are applied.

Antibiotics Classes:

- **Penicillins and cephalosporins:** Assault the cell walls of bacteria.

- **Tetracyclines and macrolides:** Prevent bacteria from producing proteins.

- **Fluoroquinolones**: Obstruct *DNA* synthesis and repair.

Appropriate Use:

✓. **Prescription:** Only when issued by a medical practitioner should an antibiotic be taken.

✓. **Complete Course:** To avoid antibiotic resistance, take the complete suggested course of therapy, even if your symptoms go better. schedule and dose: Follow the specified schedule and dose.

Resistance To Antibiotics.

Antibiotic resistance in bacteria can occur from overuse or misuse, making infections more difficult to cure.
This stresses how vital it is to use antibiotics carefully.

Adverse Reactions:

<> **Allergic Reactions**: Certain antibiotics may induce allergies in certain people.

<> **Disruption of Normal Flora:**
Antibiotics have the ability to change
the body's good flora, which can
result in diseases like diarrhea.

Use of Antiseptics and Disinfectants:

<> **Preparing the skin:** This
minimizes the likelihood of infection
prior to surgery.

Used on wounds to limit the growth of bacteria.

Problems and Upcoming Changes:

<> **Antibiotic Development:** Finding novel antibiotics is tough, and the issue of antibiotic resistance is growing more and more important.

<> **Investigation into Alternatives:** Continued investigation into

replacement treatments such as immunotherapy and phage therapy.

It is necessary to know the multiple uses and probable downsides of antibacterials in order to assist in efficient treatment and prevent the establishment of antibiotic-resistant strains.

Chapter 6: **How To Use Natural Remedies To Combat Infections.**

Supporting the immune system to fight infections can be performed with the use of natural remedies. *All you need to know is this:*

✓. **Hydration:** Drinking adequate water boosts general health and aids in the elimination of contaminants.

Eat a diet heavy in minerals *(zinc)*, vitamins *(C, D, and E),* and antioxidants. Citrus fruits, leafy greens, nuts, and seeds are a few examples.

✓. **Garlic:** Added to food or taken as a supplement, garlic is well-known for its antimicrobial characteristics.

How to apply:

Crush and consume two to three raw garlic cloves each day to enhance your defenses against bacterial and other infections.

Additionally, you can add freshly crushed garlic to your soups, salads, and drinks.

Curcumin, which has anti-inflammatory and antibacterial properties, is present in turmeric. For better absorption, combine black pepper and turmeric.

For ages, it has been extensively utilized in Chinese and Ayurvedic medicinal systems to treat a wide range of ailments. Because of its powerful antibacterial and anti-inflammatory qualities, it is particularly beneficial in treating a number of bacterial infections.

It can even be applied topically to treat staph infections brought on by antibiotic-resistant bacterial strains like *MRSA*.

Moreover, turmeric can be used topically to aid in the faster healing of skin illnesses and wounds.

This antibacterial agent helps prevent infection of the wounded skin when applied to an open wound.

Additionally, you can enhance your body's defenses against infection by taking turmeric internally.

How to apply:

Apply a tiny amount of organic honey and turmeric to the affected region to aid in the healing of wounds and the eradication of skin infections.

To improve immunity, one tablespoon of turmeric powder and five to six tablespoons of honey should be blended, then kept in an airtight container. Take one-half teaspoon of this combination twice daily. Asking our doctor to start you on a turmeric supplement is another alternative.

✓. **Ginger contains antioxidants and anti-inflammatory**

characteristics. Make ginger tea or incorporate it into cuisine.

Ginger prevents and cures a wide spectrum of bacterial illnesses by acting as a natural antibiotic.

Particularly potent against bacteria found in food, such as salmonella, is fresh ginger. Moreover, it possesses antimicrobial characteristics that protect against periodontal and respiratory disorders.

How to apply:

In order to avoid bacterial infections:

Grate a one-inch piece of fresh ginger
and simmer it for ten minutes in one
and a half cups of water. Pour the
liquid through a filter into a cup, taste
and add honey and lemon juice, and
enjoy your daily cup of ginger tea.
As much as possible, utilize fresh or
dried ginger in your dishes.
To take supplements containing
ginger, speak with your doctor.

Honey has specific antibacterial characteristics that prevent infections on various levels and impede the development of bacterial resistance.

Honey's therapeutic qualities can be connected to its acidic composition, natural sugar content, hydrogen peroxide, and polyphenolic antioxidant components.

Therefore, unlike conventional antibiotics, honey employs a variety of techniques to launch a multi pronged attack against infection-causing germs without interfering with the necessary growth of good bacteria.

This preserves your gut bacteria in good health and prevents you from experiencing the unneeded stomach discomfort that comes with taking antibiotics. Furthermore, healthy bacteria are important to protect your immunity and general well-being.

Additionally, honey can destroy bacterial strains that have evolved resistance to several antibiotic treatments; yet, this treatment is most effective when paired with an antibiotic. Honey has an extra benefit over conventional antibiotics in that it works well against viruses and has no unnecessary side effects.

How to apply:

To increase your immunity when you're sick, eat equal parts honey and cinnamon once a day.

Another simple option to include honey in your daily diet and benefit from its health advantages is to use it as a sweetener for tea, smoothies, and juices.

Probiotics boost immunity by maintaining gut health. Fermented foods, kefir, and yogurt are excellent sources.

Echinacea could aid in immune system stimulation. accessible as herbal drinks or supplements.

Certain essential oils, such as tea tree oil, possess antimicrobial characteristics. Use diluted products for topical therapy or in diffusers.

Supplemental vitamin C boosts immunity. If you don't consume enough food, think about taking supplements.

Rest and sleep are vital for healing because they allow the body to recover itself.

Frequent exercise increases the immune response and general health.

A variety of herbs, spices, flowers, or other plant components are infused into hot water to create herbal teas.

Herbal teas don't contain caffeine like true teas do, which are manufactured from the Camellia plant. They are valued for their variety of tastes, relaxing characteristics, and possibly health perks.

Herbal Tea Types.

Famous for its stimulating flavor and digestive effects, peppermint tea.

Tea brewed with chamomile is often used to improve serenity and enhance sleep.
Ginger tea is regarded for its probable anti-inflammatory qualities and has a spicy flavor.

Aromatic and relaxing, lavender tea is widely used to reduce stress.
Bright and tart, hibiscus tea is said to offer antioxidant characteristics.
Echinacea tea is supposed to enhance the defenses against illness, especially in the winter.

✓ **Tea with Turmeric:** This tea contains turmeric, an

anti-inflammatory spice that's usually blended with other herbs.

✓ **Nettle Tea:** Known for its potential health advantages, this tea is rich in vitamins and minerals.

Advantages for Health:

✓ **Antioxidant Properties:** Antioxidants can help avoid oxidative stress and are present in a variety of herbal teas.

✓ **Digestive Aid:** Teas with ginger and peppermint are well-liked for easing unsettled stomachs.

✓. **Stress Reduction:** Calming herbs like chamomile, lavender, and others can aid in lowering tension and fostering relaxation.

✓. **Immune Support:** The immune system is thought to be supported by several herbal drinks, such as echinacea.

✓. **Anti-Inflammatory Effects:**
Anti-inflammatory capabilities are connected to ginger and turmeric teas.

Brewing Advice.

Water temperature: 180–212°F (82–100°C), depending on the herb. *Steeping Time:* 5 to 10 minutes on average, but may take longer depending on the herbs used.

✓. **Serving size:** one to two tablespoons of dried herbs for every eight ounces of water.

Taking into account

✓. **Pregnancy:** Speak with a healthcare provider before ingesting any herbal teas, as some may not be safe.

✓. **Allergies:** People who are allergic to plants should take caution when taking various herbal medicines.

Herbal teas are a popular choice for consumers looking for caffeine-free tea alternatives because they come in a range of flavors and may have health advantages.

Acetic acid, contained in apple cider vinegar, may aid in the elimination of harmful microorganisms. Consume in moderation after diluting.

✓. **Remain Stress-Free:** Prolonged stress lowers immunity. Use relaxation strategies such as deep breathing exercises or meditation.

Recall that although natural therapies can support medical interventions, severe infections or chronic symptoms should always be examined by a physician. *These instructions should not be used in place of competent medical advice.*

Conclusion.

To sum up, the discovery of the herbal antibiotics revolution is a huge step toward merging old knowledge with contemporary science, and it presents potential substitutes for existing pharmaceuticals.

Respecting the rights and knowledge of indigenous populations, we must approach this transition with cultural sensitivity and ethical considerations. Through the emphasis of informed consent, benefit sharing, cultural sensitivity, and long-term relationships, I guarantee that the invention and application of herbal antibiotics are carried out in an amicable, accountable, and complete way. This policy not only protects traditional wisdom but also stimulates true cooperation and opens the path to just and sustainable healthcare solutions.

About

Spend at least three (3) hours daily by reading these works and considering these important theories.

Information: Learning & Research.

Well-being: working, learning, building gold.

Crowd: *system administration and building my clans*

Character: Reflection, intercession and knowing my self outcome *(in business and life, both in Christendom).*

Thank You Once More for Reading
This Book and, Above All, Thank You
for Buying It.

Do have a wonderful life!